My Sister Has Diabetes
and How That Makes Me Feel

by
Grace Rooney

Illustrated by
Michele Pensa

All proceeds from the sale of <u>My Sister Has Diabetes</u>
will benefit Support for Siblings, 501(c)(3).

Do you know someone else who would like this book?
Additional copies may be purchased through
Amazon.com

We'd love to hear from you! Email us at
SupportForSiblings@aol.com

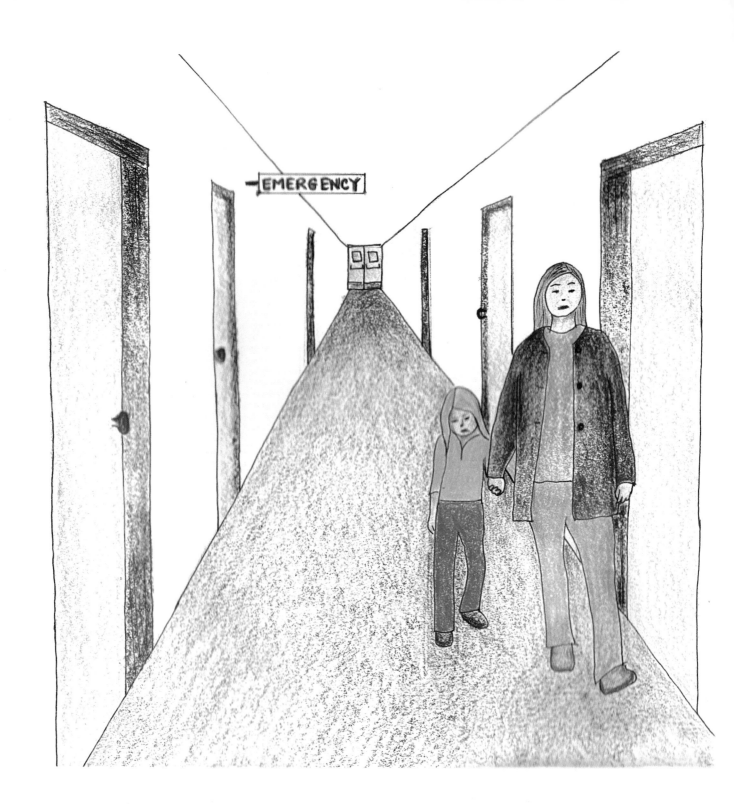

My name is Grace. When I was two years old, my big sister, Paige, got really sick. Mom, Dad, and I took her to the hospital. The doctor told us that she had Type 1 Diabetes. My mom started to cry a lot. My dad cried a little too. My aunt came to the hospital to pick me up. Mom, Dad, and Paige all stayed together without me.

That made me feel like crying.

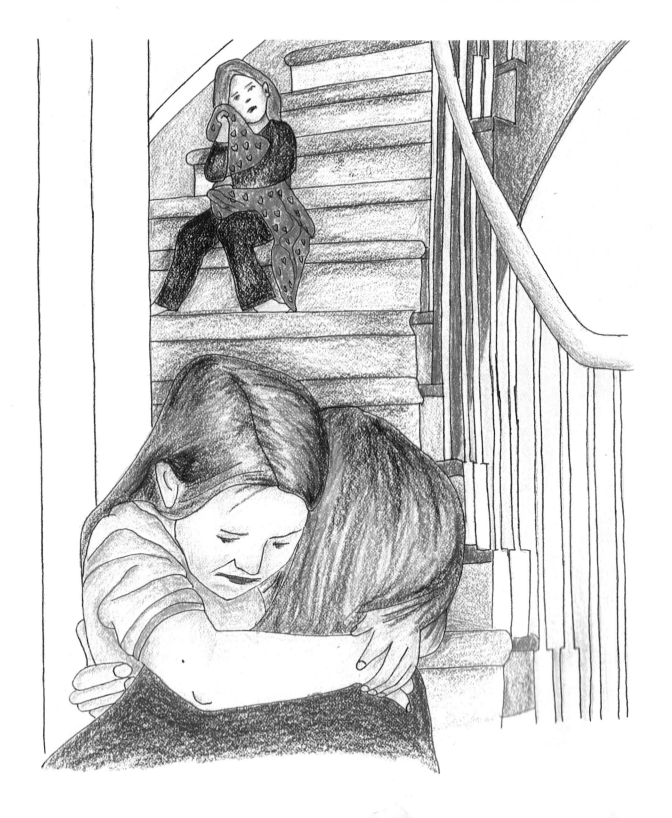

Mom and Dad learned that they would have to give my sister shots and poke her fingers every day. They said it was to keep her healthy, but Paige hated it. When I watched, it seemed like my parents were hurting my sister.

That made me feel scared.

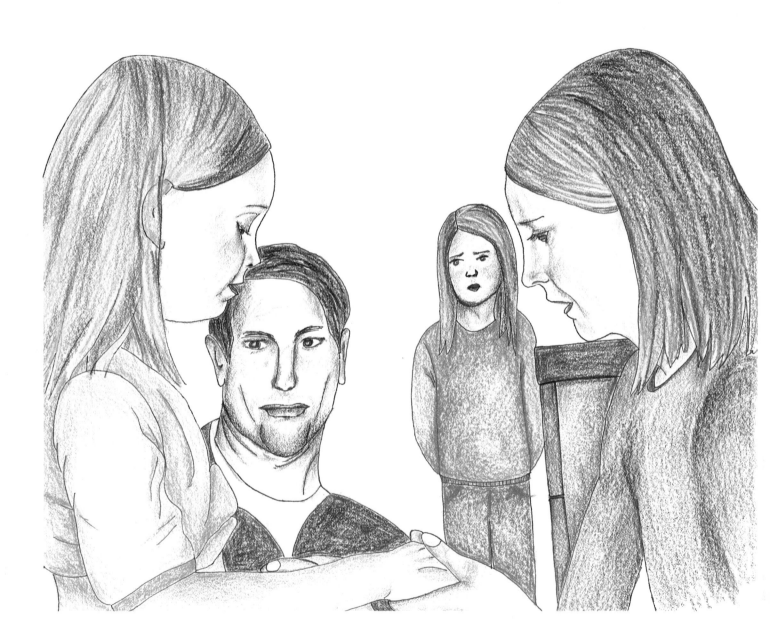

These days, my sister uses an insulin pump instead of getting shots. Now she has to get her pump site changed. It hurts Paige just like getting a shot because they still have to stick a needle in her.

When my sister gets her pump site changed, she likes to have both my mom and dad hold her hands when the needle goes in.

That makes me feel left out.

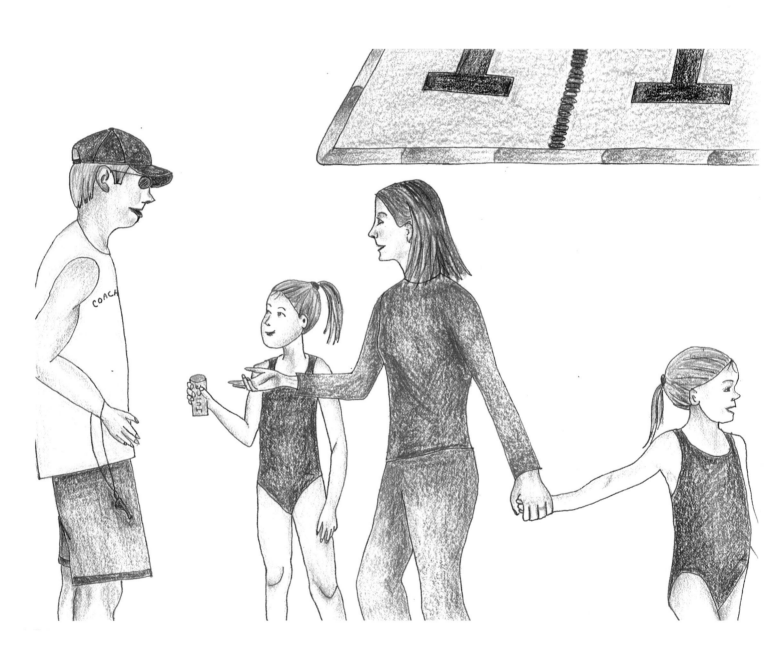

Whenever we go someplace, people ask a bunch of questions about my sister's diabetes. My mom has to explain to Paige's teachers, coaches, and babysitters how to take care of her. It takes so long, and I get tired of waiting.

That makes me feel frustrated.

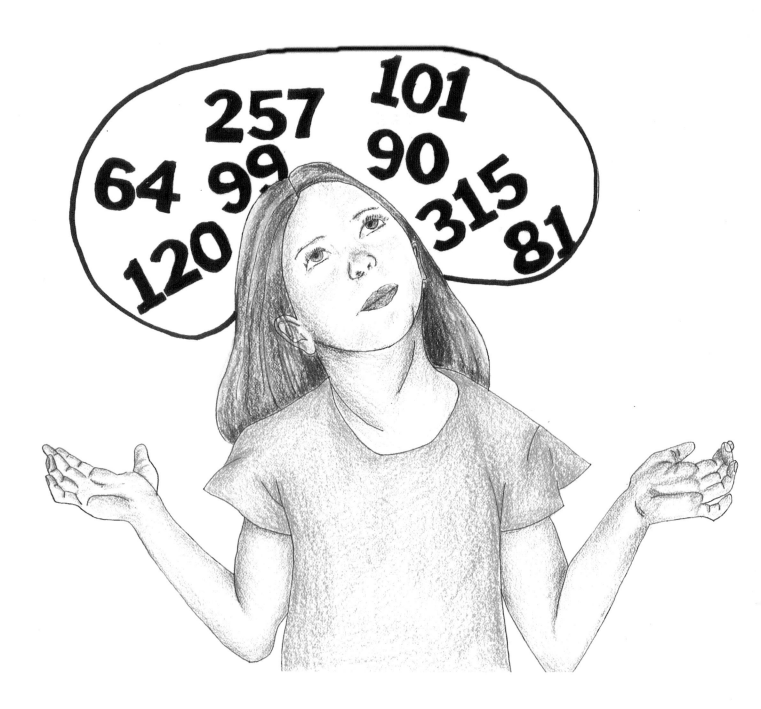

When Paige is low, she has to eat candy. When she is high, she can't. Sometimes Mom and Dad make her drink juice even if she doesn't want any. Sometimes she can't eat anything sweet. Mom and Dad say things like "she's 64" or "315" or "101".

That makes me feel confused.

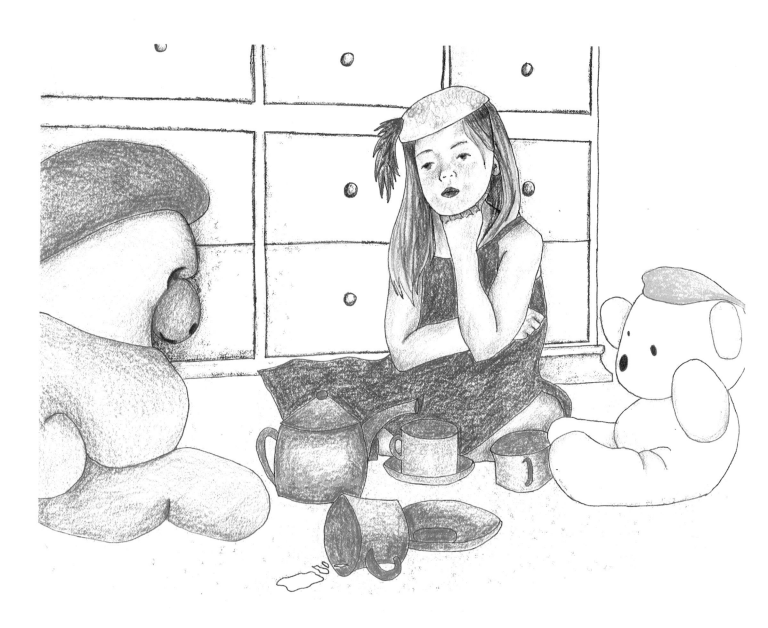

Sometimes when Paige is low, she acts mean to me. She gets mad and grumpy even if we're having fun playing. Mom and Dad say it's not my fault and that Paige can't help it. We have to stop whatever we're doing so she can test her blood sugar and have a snack.

That makes me feel sad.

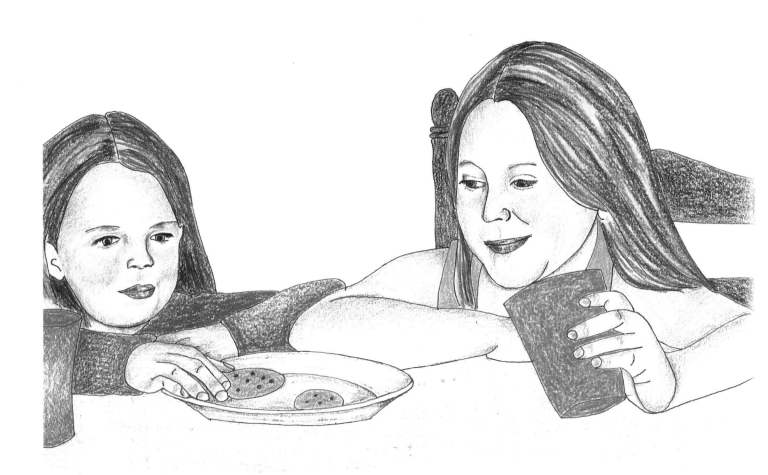

If Paige is low before dinner, then we get to have dessert first. If she's low before we go to sleep, we'll have a juice and cookie party at bedtime.

That makes me feel excited.

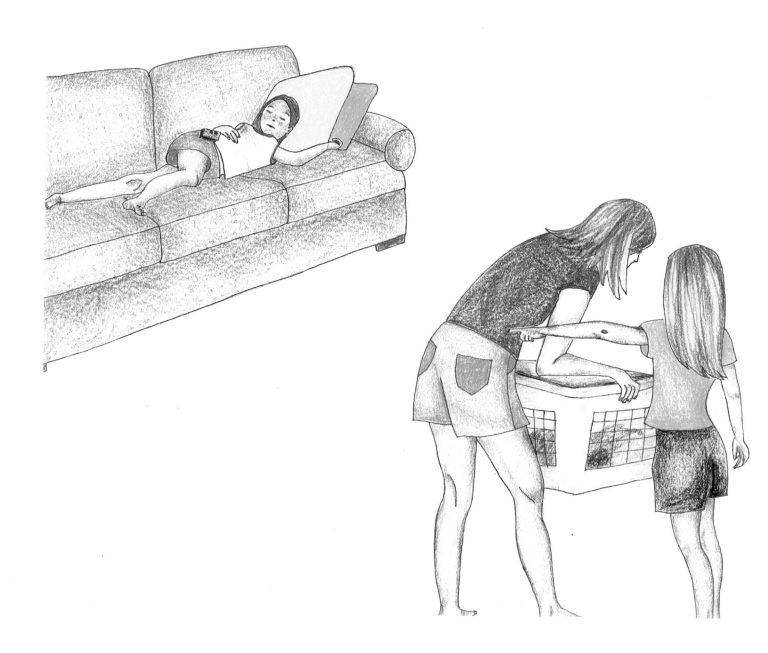

Sometimes I can tell if Paige's blood sugar is dropping even before she can feel it herself. Then I find my mom or dad and say, "I think Paige is low." I'm almost always right. I know that I am helping my sister stay healthy.

That makes me feel proud.

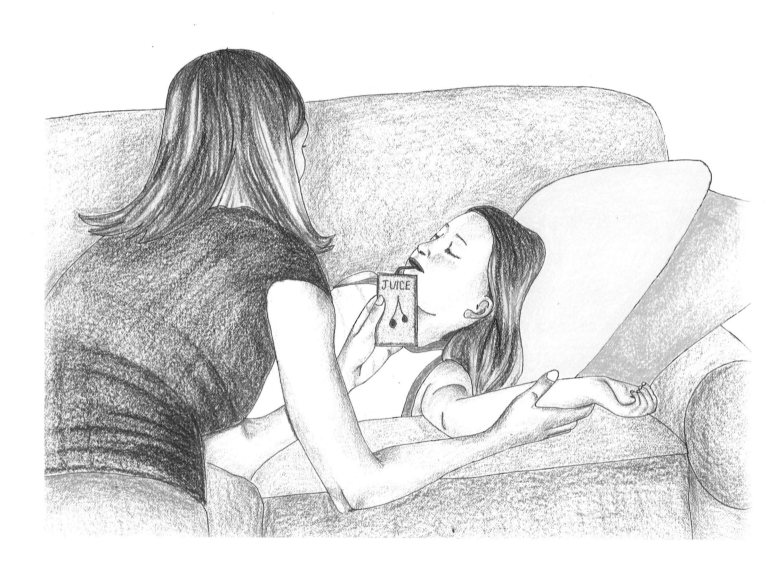

If Paige gets so low that she falls asleep during the day, Mom rushes to test her blood sugar and has to give her juice right away.

That makes me feel worried.

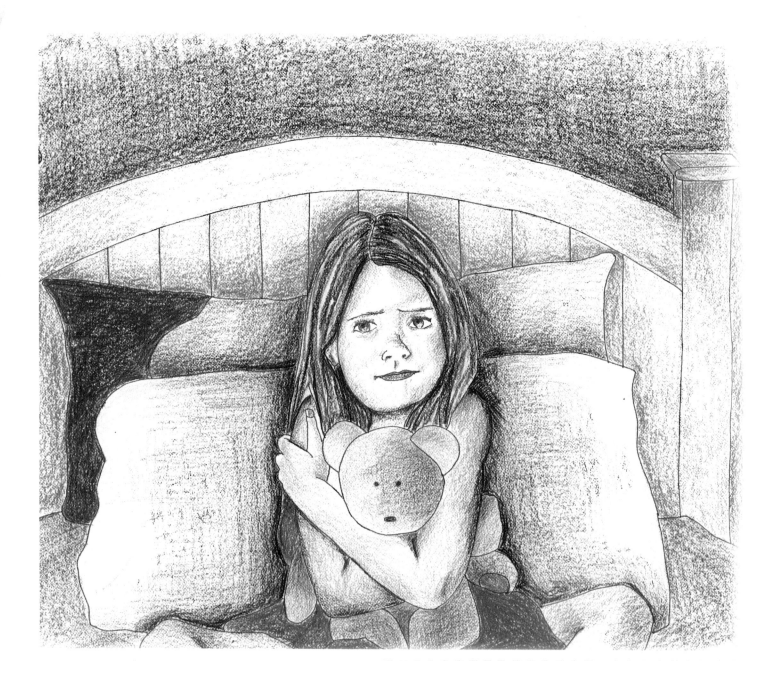

Once I had a really bad dream. In my dream my sister and I were home alone. Paige fell asleep and I couldn't wake her up. I had to call 911 and the firemen came and took her to the hospital.

That made me feel terrified.

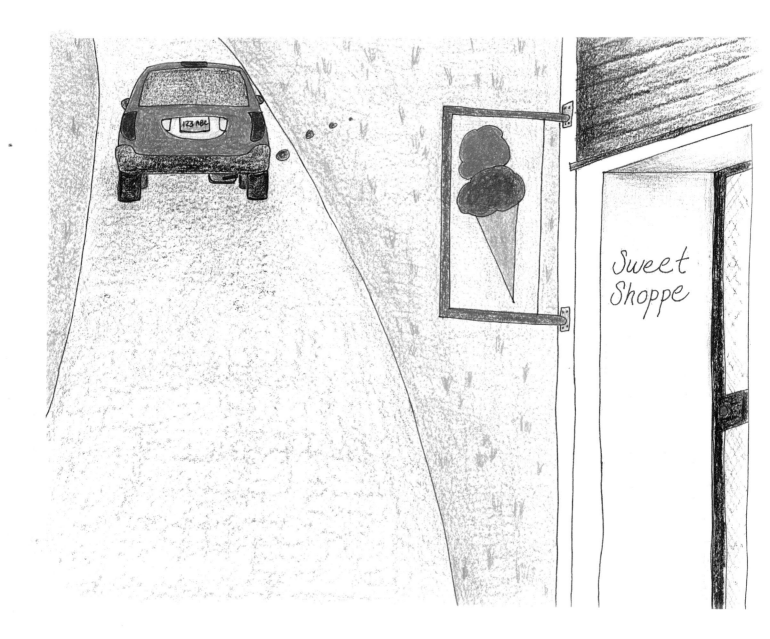

One time my mom said we could have ice cream. But when we got to the shop, Paige tested her blood sugar, and she was really high. My mom promised we'd get ice cream another day.

That made me feel disappointed.

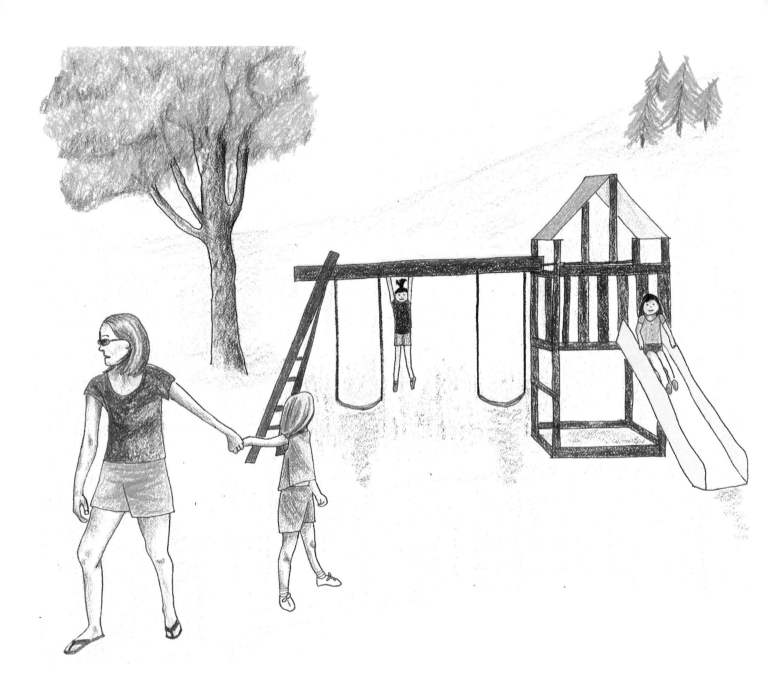

Another day my mom and I were at the park. The school nurse called because Paige's blood sugar was really high. We had to go and pick her up right away so Mom could change her pump site. I didn't even get to swing.

That made me feel mad.

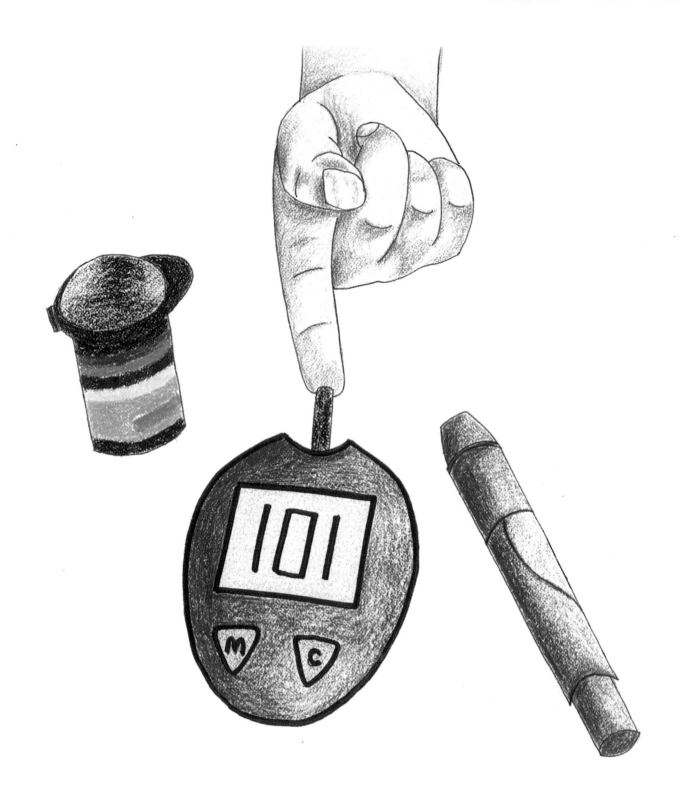

Whenever Paige tests her blood sugar, I wonder will she be high? Will she be low? Most of the time, she's in the target range.

That makes me feel relieved.

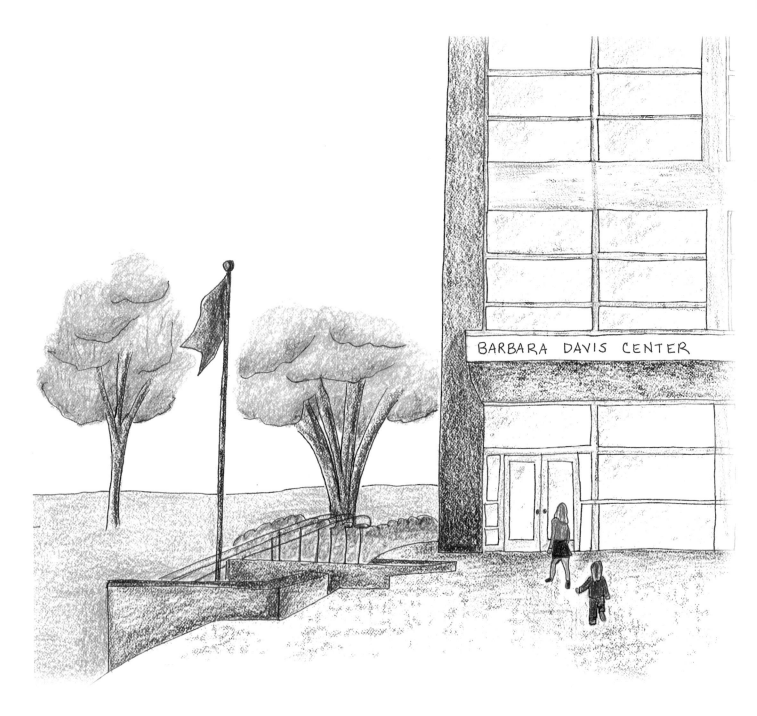

I have to go to the TEDDY (The Environmental Determinants of Diabetes in the Young) study, so the doctors can see if I am going to get diabetes too. They say that I probably won't.

That makes me feel reassured.

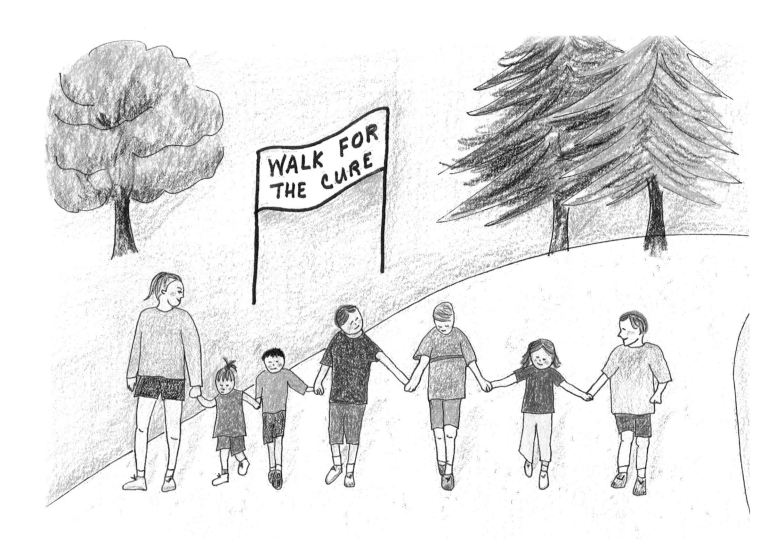

I want my sister to have a healthy life so she can always be with me. I think about how some day there may be a cure. My cousins, friends, and I raise money every year so doctors can figure out how to make diabetes go away.

That makes me feel hopeful.

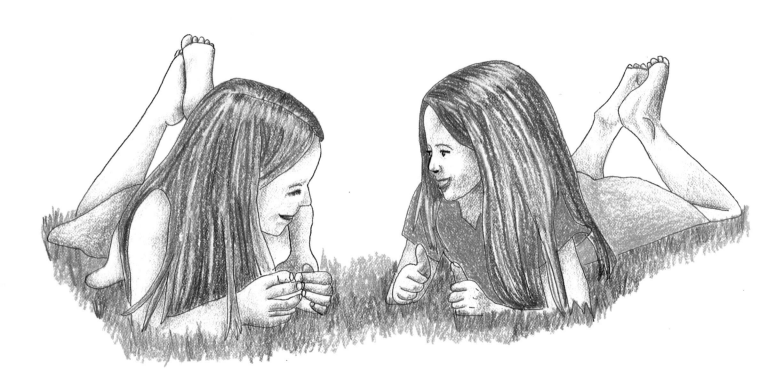

My sister has Type 1 Diabetes, and I have a lot of different feelings about it. Most of the time, no one asks about my feelings because Paige is the one who has diabetes. But it seems like our whole family has diabetes because it changed all of our lives. I hope other kids who have a sister or brother or cousin or friend or mother or father with diabetes will feel better after reading this book.

That will make me feel happy.

Printed in Great Britain
by Amazon